Extending Strong

A Guide for Over 50s Adaptability:

Change Your Wellbeing, Upgrade Portability, and Embrace Life's Next Part with Certainty

BY

Peace Monaco

CONTENTS

INTRODUCTION

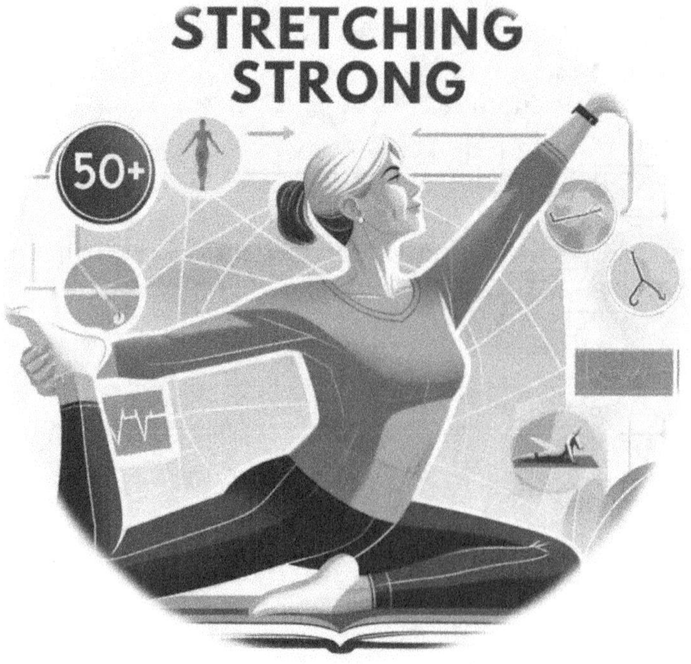

"Life is a journey filled with twists, turns, and unexpected detours. As we navigate the path of aging, it's easy to feel overwhelmed by the changes that come with each passing year. But what if I told you that turning 50 isn't the end of the road—it's just the beginning of a new chapter filled with vitality, strength, and endless possibilities?"

Welcome to "Stretching Strong: A Roadmap for Over-50s Flexibility," where we embark on a transformative journey of health, vitality, and self-discovery. In this book, we'll explore the power of flexibility as a cornerstone of post-50 wellness, providing you with the tools and knowledge to embrace life's next chapter with confidence and resilience.

Setting the Scene: Shifting the Paradigm of Aging

For far too long, society has perpetuated the myth that aging inevitably leads to decline—a narrative that paints a bleak picture of the second half of life. But the truth is far more empowering. With advances in healthcare, nutrition, and fitness, we have the opportunity to redefine what it means to age gracefully and vibrantly.

In "Stretching Strong," we challenge the conventional wisdom of aging, shifting the paradigm from one of decline to one of empowered vitality. Rather than resigning ourselves to the limitations imposed by age, we embrace the potential for growth, resilience, and fulfillment that comes with each passing year.

The Multifaceted Benefits of Flexibility: Beyond Just Touching Your Toes

Flexibility is often misunderstood as simply the ability to touch your toes or perform a split. However, its benefits extend far beyond mere physical prowess. In "Stretching Strong," we explore the multifaceted benefits of flexibility, from improved mobility and posture to enhanced mental well-being and resilience.

Through a combination of dynamic exercises, targeted stretches, and mindfulness techniques, we'll unlock the transformative power of flexibility in all areas of life. Whether you're looking to prevent injury, alleviate pain, or simply feel more confident and energized, this book offers a comprehensive roadmap to help you achieve your goals.

Your Personalized Roadmap to "Stretching Strong"

At the heart of "Stretching Strong" lies your personalized roadmap to optimal health and vitality over 50. Drawing on the latest research in physiology, biomechanics, and psychology, we'll guide you through a step-by-step journey of self-discovery and empowerment.

From establishing your baseline flexibility to developing a sustainable stretching routine, each chapter is designed to provide you with actionable insights and practical strategies for success. Whether you're a seasoned athlete or new to the world of fitness, "Stretching Strong" offers something for everyone, empowering you to unlock your full potential and embrace life's next chapter with confidence and resilience.

Conclusion: Embrace the Journey Ahead

As we embark on this journey together, remember that the road to optimal health and vitality is not always smooth or linear. There will be challenges, setbacks, and moments of doubt along the way. But with perseverance, determination, and a willingness to embrace change, you can overcome any obstacle and achieve the vibrant, fulfilling life you deserve.

So, are you ready to embark on the journey of a lifetime? Are you ready to stretch strong and embrace the limitless potential that comes with age? If so, then let's begin. Your journey to wellness over 50 starts now.

Part 1:
Embracing Change
& Redefining
Strength

Chapter 01

Flexibility for Life After 50

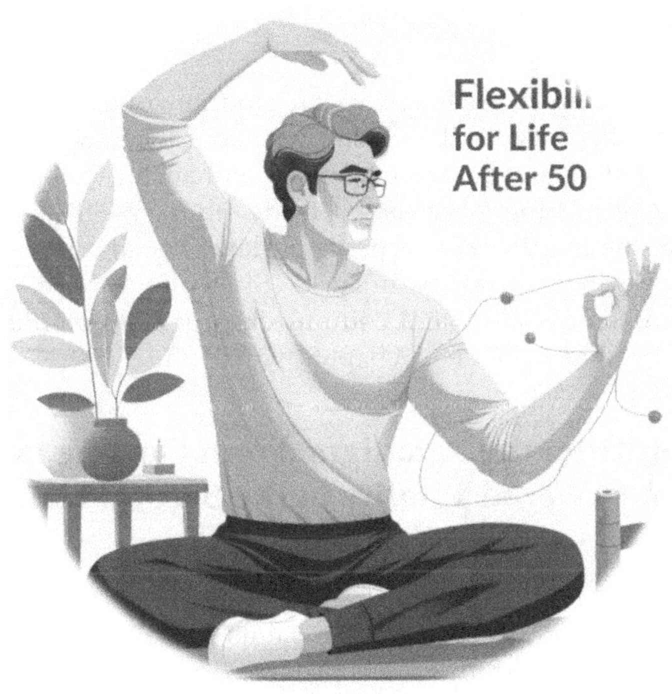

"Age is no barrier when it comes to flexibility. In fact, it's the cornerstone of post-50 wellness, unlocking a vitality you never knew you had."

As we journey through life, our bodies inevitably undergo changes. We may notice a little stiffness here, a bit of reduced mobility there, and perhaps even a sense of apprehension about what lies ahead. But what if I told you that these changes don't have to signify a decline? What if, instead, they could be the catalyst for a redefinition of strength and vitality in the second half of life?

In this chapter, we'll embark on a journey of discovery, exploring why flexibility isn't just about touching your toes — it's about embracing change, enhancing mobility, and reclaiming your sense of adventure. We'll delve into the multifaceted benefits of flexibility and unveil your personalized roadmap to "Stretching Strong," a guide designed to help you unlock your full potential and embrace life's next chapter with confidence.

Shifting the Paradigm: From Decline to Empowered Vitality in the Second Half of Life

It's no secret that society often paints a bleak picture of aging — a narrative characterized by decline, limitations, and a dwindling sense of vitality. But what if we challenge this narrative? What if we refuse to accept that getting older means settling for less?

The truth is, the second half of life presents us with an opportunity — an opportunity to redefine what it means to be strong, vibrant, and resilient. Instead of viewing aging as a downward spiral, we can choose to see it as a journey of growth, wisdom, and newfound freedom. By shifting our paradigm from one of decline to one of empowered vitality, we open ourselves up to a world of possibilities, where age is not a barrier, but a badge of honor.

The Multifaceted Benefits of Flexibility: Beyond Just Touching Your Toes

When we think of flexibility, we often envision contortionists and gymnasts bending and twisting their bodies in extraordinary ways. But flexibility is not just reserved for the elite few — it's a fundamental aspect of human movement that impacts every aspect of our lives.

From improving posture and reducing the risk of injury to enhancing athletic performance and relieving stress, the benefits of flexibility are far-reaching and profound. By prioritizing flexibility in our wellness routines, we can increase our range of motion, improve joint health, and cultivate a sense of ease and fluidity in our bodies.

Enhanced Mobility for an Active Lifestyle: From Independent Living to Adventurous Pursuits

Mobility is the key to independence, allowing us to navigate the world with confidence and grace. Whether it's bending down to tie our shoes, reaching for a high shelf, or embarking on a new outdoor adventure, mobility plays a crucial role in every aspect of daily life.

By prioritizing flexibility and mobility in our wellness routines, we can ensure that we remain active, engaged, and independent well into our golden years. Whether you're a seasoned athlete or a weekend warrior, incorporating stretching and mobility exercises into your daily routine can help you maintain optimal function and vitality.

Your Personalized Roadmap to "Stretching Strong": A Step-by-Step Guide to Unlocking Your Full Potential

Embarking on a journey of transformation requires a roadmap—a clear and actionable plan that guides us toward our goals. In "Stretching Strong," we'll provide you with a step-by-step guide to unlocking your full potential, tailored specifically to your needs and preferences.

From identifying your current level of flexibility to setting realistic goals and creating a personalized stretching routine, our roadmap will empower you to take control of your health and embrace life's next chapter with confidence. Whether you're looking to improve your mobility, reduce pain and stiffness, or simply enhance your overall quality of life, "Stretching

Strong" will be your trusted companion every step of the way.

In the chapters that follow, we'll delve deeper into the science of flexibility, explore practical strategies for integrating stretching into your daily routine, and celebrate the transformative power of movement at any age. So let's embark on this journey together, as we discover the joy of "Stretching Strong" and unlock the boundless potential that lies within each and every one of us.

Chapter 02

Redefining Strength Over 50

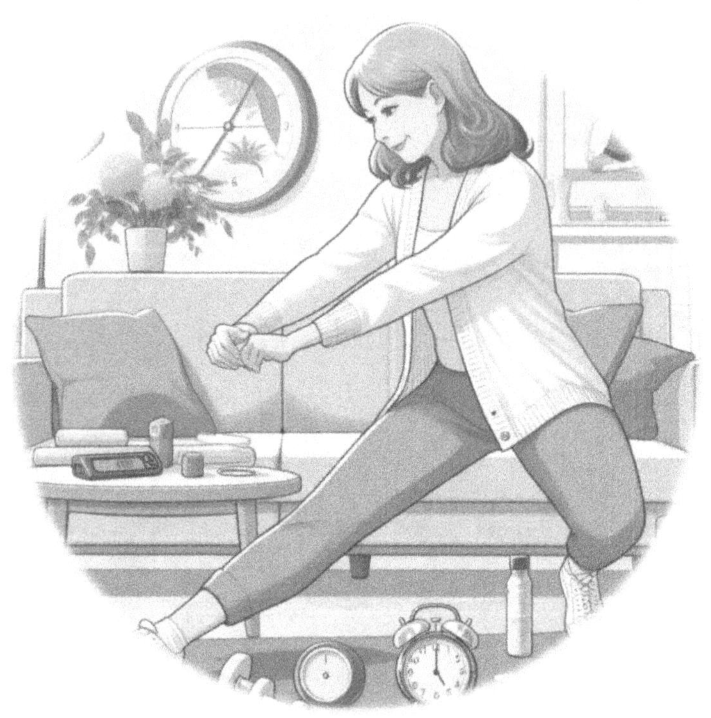

As we age, the notion of strength takes on a new meaning. It's no longer just about how much weight we can lift or how many push-ups we can do. Instead, it's about building functional capacity — the ability to perform everyday movements with ease and confidence, ensuring sustained independence and vitality well into our golden years.

In this chapter, we'll redefine strength after 50, exploring the importance of functional strength training, the role of the core in stability and support, and practical exercises for real-world application. Along the way, we'll debunk common myths surrounding strength training, proving that it's not just for bodybuilders — it's for everyone who wants to live life to the fullest.

Functional Strength Training: Everyday Movements for Sustained Independence

Functional strength training focuses on movements that mimic activities of daily living, such as bending, lifting, reaching, and squatting. By training these movements, we not only build strength in the muscles involved but also improve balance, coordination, and proprioception — the body's awareness of its position in space.

Unlike traditional strength training, which often emphasizes isolated muscle groups and heavy weights, functional strength training prioritizes movement quality and functionality. This approach ensures that our bodies are equipped to handle the demands of everyday life, reducing the risk of injury and enhancing our overall quality of life.

The Core: The Foundation for Stability and Support in All Activities

When it comes to building strength after 50, the core is often overlooked—but it shouldn't be. The core muscles, which include the abdominals, obliques, and lower back, serve as the foundation for stability and support in virtually every movement we make.

A strong core not only improves posture and balance but also reduces the risk of back pain and injury. By incorporating core-strengthening exercises into our routine, such as planks, bridges, and rotational movements, we can enhance our functional capacity and maintain optimal stability and support as we age.

Strength Training Beyond the Gym: Exercises for Real-World Application

Strength training doesn't have to be confined to the walls of a gym. In fact, some of the most effective exercises for building functional capacity can be performed in the comfort of your own home or even outdoors.

Bodyweight exercises, such as squats, lunges, and push-ups, require no equipment and can be modified to suit any fitness level. Resistance bands, stability balls, and even everyday household items can also be used to add variety and intensity to your workouts.

By incorporating strength training exercises into your daily routine, you'll not only build muscle and improve strength but also enhance your ability to perform everyday tasks with ease and confidence.

Debunking Strength Training Myths: It's Not Just for Bodybuilders, It's for Everyone

Strength training has long been associated with bodybuilders and athletes, leading many people to believe that it's not suitable for the average person, especially as they age. But nothing could be further from the truth.

In reality, strength training is beneficial for people of all ages and fitness levels. It helps preserve lean muscle mass, boost metabolism, and improve bone density, reducing the risk of osteoporosis and age-related muscle loss.

Furthermore, strength training can enhance functional capacity, making everyday activities easier and more enjoyable. So don't let misconceptions hold you back—embrace the power of strength training and unlock your full potential at any age.

As we've explored in this chapter, strength after 50 is about more than just building muscle—it's about building functional capacity for a life of sustained independence and vitality. By prioritizing functional strength training, focusing on the core, and incorporating real-world exercises into your routine, you can redefine what it means to be strong and embrace life's next chapter with confidence and vigor.

Chapter 03

The Importance of Flexibility: More Than Staying Limber

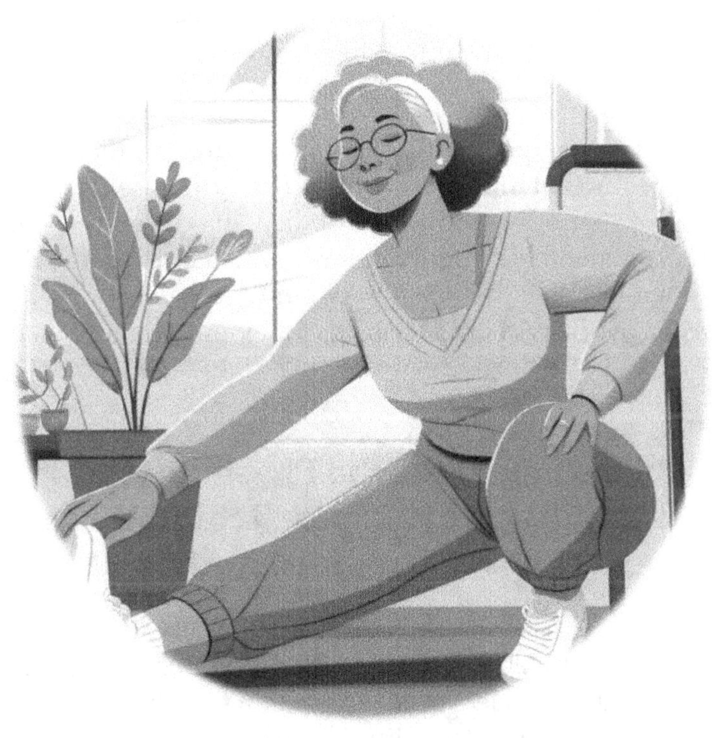

*"Flexibility isn't just about touching your toes —
it's about preserving vitality, managing pain,
preventing falls, and boosting overall well-being
well into your golden years."*

Flexibility is often viewed as a marker of youth—a trait associated with gymnasts and dancers rather than mature adults. However, as we age, the importance of flexibility becomes increasingly apparent. It's not just about staying limber; it's about preserving vitality, managing pain, preventing falls, and boosting overall well-being well into our golden years.

In this chapter, we'll delve into the multifaceted importance of flexibility in mature adults, exploring the physiology behind flexibility, its role in pain management, fall prevention, and circulation. By understanding the science behind flexibility and its profound impact on our health and well-being, we can unlock the key to a life of vitality and independence.

Understanding the Physiology of Flexibility: The Science Behind What Happens to Our Bodies After 50

Flexibility is determined by a combination of factors, including muscle elasticity, joint mobility, and connective tissue flexibility. As we age, these factors naturally decline due to changes in collagen production, joint lubrication, and muscle mass.

However, aging doesn't have to mean a loss of flexibility. By incorporating regular stretching and mobility exercises into our routine, we can counteract these age-related changes and maintain or even improve our flexibility well into our later years.

Understanding the physiology of flexibility empowers us to take proactive steps to preserve our mobility and independence as we age. By prioritizing flexibility in our wellness routines, we can mitigate the effects of aging and enjoy a higher quality of life for years to come.

Flexibility and Pain Management: Improving Flexibility as a Strategy for Reducing Discomfort

Chronic pain is a common companion for many mature adults, often stemming from conditions such as arthritis, back pain, and joint stiffness. While pain medications may offer temporary relief, they often come with unwanted side effects and fail to address the underlying cause of the pain.

Flexibility plays a crucial role in pain management, as tight muscles and stiff joints can exacerbate discomfort and limit mobility. By improving flexibility through regular stretching and mobility exercises, we can alleviate tension, reduce inflammation, and promote healing in the affected areas.

Additionally, increased flexibility can help correct imbalances in the body, improve posture, and reduce the risk of injury—all of which contribute to long-term pain relief and improved quality of life.

Fall Prevention Through Enhanced Mobility: Reducing the Risk of Injury and Maintaining Independence

Falls are a leading cause of injury and loss of independence among mature adults, often resulting in fractures, sprains, and other serious injuries. As we age, changes in balance, coordination, and reaction time can increase the risk of falls, making fall prevention a critical component of healthy aging.

Flexibility plays a key role in fall prevention by improving mobility, agility, and proprioception—the body's ability to sense its position in space. By incorporating stretching and mobility exercises into our routine, we can enhance our balance, coordination, and reaction time, reducing the risk of falls and maintaining our independence for longer.

Flexibility and Improved Circulation: Boosting Energy Levels and Overall Well-being

Good circulation is essential for delivering oxygen and nutrients to the cells, removing waste products, and maintaining overall health and well-being. Poor circulation, on the other hand, can lead to fatigue, muscle cramps, and a host of other health issues.

Flexibility plays a crucial role in circulation by promoting blood flow to the muscles, joints, and tissues. By stretching and mobilizing the body, we can enhance circulation, improve oxygenation, and boost energy levels throughout the day.

Additionally, increased flexibility can help reduce tension and stiffness in the muscles, allowing for greater freedom of movement and a heightened sense of vitality. By prioritizing flexibility in our wellness routines, we can optimize circulation and enjoy a higher level of energy and well-being well into our later years.

In summary, flexibility is more than just staying limber—it's a key component of healthy aging that impacts every aspect of our lives. By understanding the physiology of flexibility and its profound effects on pain management, fall prevention, and circulation, we can unlock the key to a life of vitality, independence, and well-being well into our golden years.

Part 2:
Building a Strong Foundation

Chapter 04

Body Awareness:
Find Your Baseline

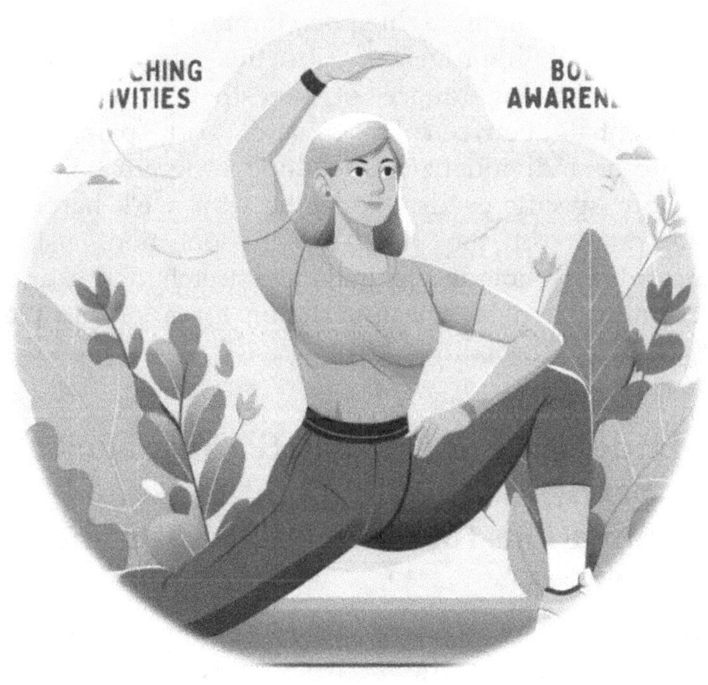

"Flexibility begins with awareness. By tuning into your body, identifying limitations, and understanding the difference between good and bad pain, you can create a personalized stretching program that promotes safety, effectiveness, and lasting results."

Flexibility is a journey—one that begins with body awareness. Before we can embark on the path to increased flexibility, we must first establish our baseline, identifying tight spots, limitations, and areas of potential improvement. In this chapter, we'll explore the importance of kinesthetic awareness, differentiate between "good" and "bad" pain, and create an individualized stretching program tailored to your specific needs. Along the way, we'll harness the power of the mind-body connection, using breathing techniques to enhance stretch depth and relaxation, and lay the foundation for a sustainable approach to flexibility.

Importance of Kinesthetic Awareness: Safely Identifying Tight Spots and Limitations for Personalized Routines

Kinesthetic awareness, often referred to as proprioception, is the body's ability to sense its position, movement, and orientation in space. It's what allows us to touch our toes without looking, maintain balance while walking, and perform complex movements with precision and control.

When it comes to flexibility, kinesthetic awareness plays a crucial role in identifying tight spots and limitations that may be impeding our range of motion. By tuning into our bodies and paying attention to how different movements feel, we can pinpoint areas that may need extra attention and tailor our stretching routines accordingly.

Differentiating Between "Good" and "Bad" Pain: Knowing When to Push and When to Prioritize Safety

One of the most common challenges in flexibility training is knowing when to push through discomfort and when to ease off to avoid injury. While some level of discomfort is normal during stretching, it's important to differentiate between "good" pain, which indicates productive stretching, and "bad" pain, which signals potential harm.

"Good" pain is typically described as a mild to moderate sensation of stretching or pulling in the muscles, often accompanied by a feeling of release or relief. This type of discomfort is usually transient and subsides once the stretch is released.

On the other hand, "bad" pain is sharp, stabbing, or intense in nature and may be accompanied by a sense of burning or tearing. This type of pain is a sign that you're pushing too hard and could be causing damage to the muscles, tendons, or ligaments.

By listening to our bodies and honoring the signals they send, we can strike a balance between challenging ourselves and prioritizing safety in our flexibility practice.

Creating an Individualized Stretching Program: Tailoring Stretches to Address Your Specific Needs

No two bodies are exactly alike, which is why a one-size-fits-all approach to flexibility training often falls short. To maximize results and minimize the risk of injury, it's essential to create an individualized stretching program that addresses your specific needs, goals, and limitations.

Start by assessing your current level of flexibility, paying particular attention to areas that feel tight or restricted. Then, choose stretches that target those areas while also addressing any imbalances or asymmetries in your body.

Remember to start slowly and gradually increase the intensity and duration of your stretches as your flexibility improves. And don't be afraid to experiment with different techniques and modalities to find what works best for you.

The Mind-Body Connection: Utilizing Breathing Techniques to Enhance Stretch Depth and Relaxation

The mind-body connection plays a significant role in flexibility training, influencing our ability to relax into stretches, deepen our range of motion, and cultivate a sense of calm and focus.

By incorporating breathing techniques into our stretching routine, we can enhance our flexibility practice and promote relaxation and mindfulness. Techniques such as diaphragmatic breathing, where you breathe deeply into the belly, can help release tension in the muscles and create space for deeper stretches.

As you move through your stretching routine, focus on synchronizing your breath with your movements, inhaling deeply as you prepare for a stretch and exhaling fully as you ease into it. This mindful approach not only enhances the effectiveness of the stretch but also promotes a sense of relaxation and presence in the moment.

In summary, body awareness is the cornerstone of effective flexibility training. By tuning into our bodies, differentiating between "good" and "bad" pain, creating an individualized stretching program, and harnessing the power of the mind-body connection, we can establish a sustainable foundation for flexibility that promotes safety, effectiveness, and lasting results.

Chapter 05

Sustainable Stretching Routine

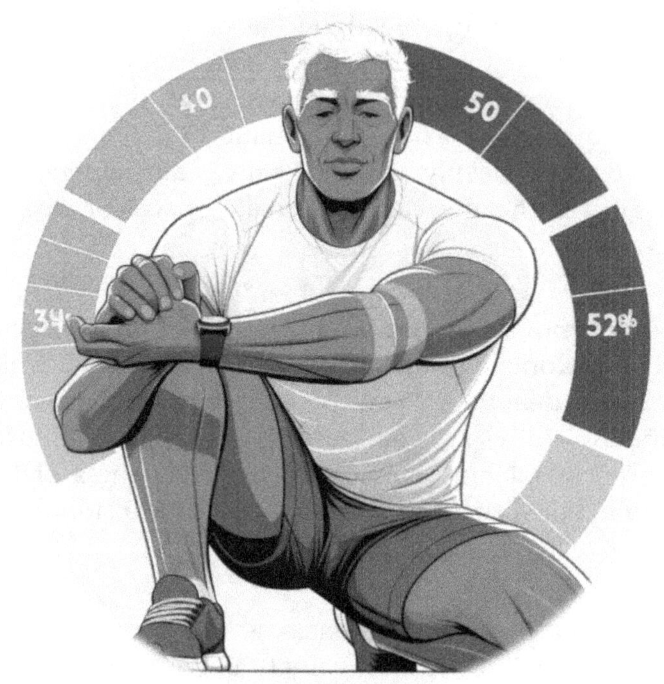

"Consistency is the key to unlocking the full potential of flexibility. By breaking the myth of 'no pain, no gain,' embracing micro-stretches, integrating stretching into daily life, and finding accountability and support, you can build a sustainable routine that yields long-term results."

Embarking on a journey to improve flexibility is not a sprint—it's a marathon. Building a sustainable stretching routine requires dedication, patience, and above all, consistency. In this chapter, we'll explore how to break the myth of "no pain, no gain," harness the power of micro-stretches, integrate stretching into your daily life, and find accountability and support to stay motivated for long-term success. By following these principles, you can build a routine that not only yields optimal results but also becomes a natural and enjoyable part of your daily routine.

Breaking the Myth of "No Pain, No Gain": Safe and Effective Stretching Practices that Yield Optimal Results

The notion that stretching should be painful to be effective is a pervasive myth—one that can lead to injury and discourage consistency in your routine. In reality, safe and effective stretching practices prioritize comfort and relaxation over pain and discomfort.

Instead of pushing yourself to the point of pain, focus on gentle, controlled movements that gradually lengthen the muscles and increase flexibility over time.

Listen to your body's signals and honor its limits, backing off if you feel any sharp or intense pain.

By adopting a mindset of ease and gentleness in your stretching practice, you'll not only reduce the risk of injury but also encourage consistency and sustainability in the long run.

The Power of Micro-Stretches: Short, Frequent Sessions Throughout the Day for Continuous Improvement

One of the biggest challenges to maintaining a stretching routine is finding the time and motivation to do it consistently. That's where the power of micro-stretches comes in.

Instead of dedicating long, grueling sessions to stretching, break your routine into shorter, more manageable chunks throughout the day. Aim for just a few minutes of stretching in the morning, during your lunch break, and before bed—no fancy equipment or dedicated workout space required.

These short, frequent sessions not only make stretching more accessible and achievable but also promote continuous improvement over time. By incorporating micro-stretches into your daily routine, you'll gradually increase flexibility, reduce stiffness, and experience the benefits of stretching in your everyday life.

Integrating Stretching into Your Daily Life: Making Stretching a Natural Part of Your Routine

Consistency is the key to long-term success in any endeavor, and stretching is no exception. To build a sustainable stretching routine, it's essential to integrate stretching into your daily life in a way that feels natural and effortless.

Find moments throughout the day when you can sneak in a quick stretch — while waiting for your coffee to brew, standing in line at the grocery store, or watching TV in the evening. By weaving stretching into the fabric of your daily routine, you'll make it a habit that requires little thought or effort to maintain.

Accountability and Support: Finding a Partner or Utilizing Resources to Stay Motivated for Long-Term Success

Even the most dedicated individuals can benefit from a little accountability and support when it comes to sticking to a stretching routine. Whether it's finding a stretching buddy to keep you accountable, joining a class or online community for support, or utilizing resources such as apps or videos for guidance and motivation, having a support system in place can make all the difference in staying consistent and committed to your routine.

Find what works best for you and lean on your support network whenever you need an extra dose of motivation or encouragement. With accountability and support by your side, you'll be well-equipped to stay on track and achieve your flexibility goals for the long haul.

In summary, developing a sustainable stretching routine is essential for achieving long-term flexibility and mobility. By breaking the myth of "no pain, no gain," embracing micro-stretches, integrating stretching into your daily life, and finding accountability and support, you can build a routine that not only yields optimal results but also becomes a natural and enjoyable part of your daily routine.

Chapter 06

Essential Stretching Gear

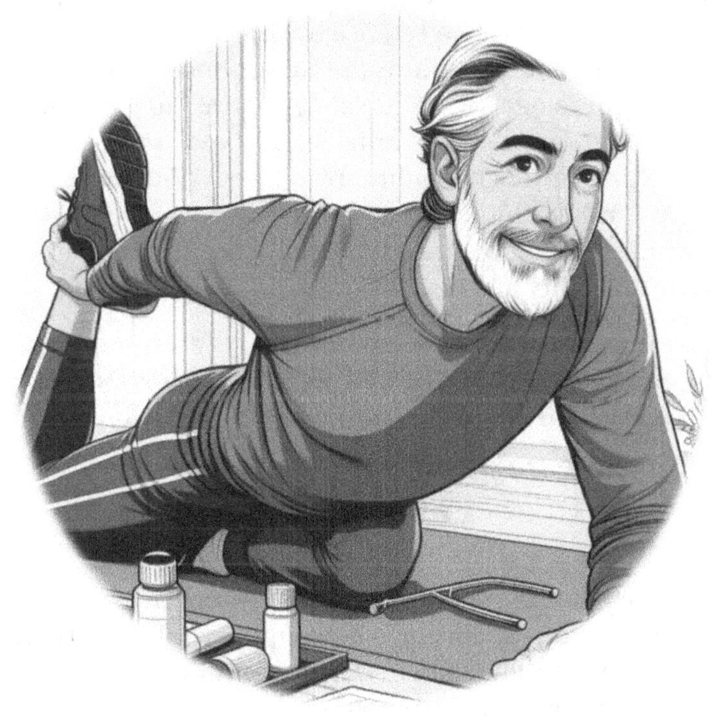

"Unlocking your flexibility potential doesn't require fancy equipment or expensive gear. By busting myths about fancy equipment, selecting the right yoga mat, maintaining flexibility on the go, and navigating stretching apps and online resources, you can optimize your practice and achieve lasting results."

When it comes to improving flexibility, the right gear can make all the difference. However, you don't need a room full of fancy equipment to optimize your practice. In this chapter, we'll debunk myths about fancy equipment, explore the importance of selecting the right yoga mat, discover how to maintain flexibility on the go, and learn how to navigate stretching apps and online resources. With the right tools and techniques at your disposal, you can optimize your practice and achieve lasting results on your flexibility journey.

Myth-Busting Fancy Equipment: Utilizing Readily Available Objects to Create an Effective Stretching Environment

Contrary to popular belief, you don't need fancy equipment or expensive gear to improve flexibility. In fact, some of the most effective stretching tools can be found right in your own home.

Everyday objects such as towels, belts, chairs, and walls can be repurposed to support your stretching practice. A towel can be used to deepen stretches or provide support during seated poses, while a belt can help extend your reach and improve alignment.

By getting creative with the objects around you, you can create an effective stretching environment without breaking the bank.

Selecting the Right Yoga Mat: Ensuring Comfort and Support for Optimal Stretching Practice

While fancy equipment isn't necessary for flexibility training, investing in a quality yoga mat can enhance your practice and provide essential comfort and support.

When selecting a yoga mat, look for one that offers adequate thickness and cushioning to protect your joints and provide stability during poses. Additionally, consider factors such as grip, durability, and eco-friendliness to ensure that your mat meets your specific needs and preferences.

A good yoga mat can make all the difference in your stretching practice, providing a supportive foundation for your poses and enhancing your overall experience.

Maintaining Flexibility on the Go: Simple Techniques to Incorporate Stretching While Traveling

Traveling doesn't have to derail your flexibility

routine. With a little creativity and planning, you can maintain your flexibility and mobility wherever your adventures take you.

Pack lightweight and portable stretching tools such as resistance bands, massage balls, or a travel-sized yoga mat to keep your practice on track while on the go. Additionally, take advantage of downtime during travel to sneak in quick stretches and mobility exercises to keep your muscles loose and limber.

By incorporating stretching into your travel routine, you can prevent stiffness, reduce muscle soreness, and ensure that you're ready to hit the ground running when you reach your destination.

Navigating Stretching Apps and Online Resources: Finding Reputable and Safe Guidance for Your Stretching Journey

In today's digital age, there's no shortage of stretching apps and online resources to guide you on your flexibility journey. However, not all resources are created equal, and it's essential to choose reputable and safe sources for guidance.

Look for apps and websites developed by certified fitness professionals or reputable organizations that provide evidence-based information and safe stretching techniques. Take the time to read reviews, check credentials, and ensure that the content aligns with your goals and abilities.

With the right stretching apps and online resources at

your fingertips, you can access expert guidance, track your progress, and stay motivated on your flexibility journey.

In summary, optimizing your flexibility practice doesn't require fancy equipment or expensive gear. By busting myths about fancy equipment, selecting the right yoga mat, maintaining flexibility on the go, and navigating stretching apps and online resources, you can optimize your practice and achieve lasting results. With the right tools and techniques at your disposal, you'll be well-equipped to unlock your flexibility potential and embrace a life of vitality and mobility.

Part 3:
The Art of Stretching

Chapter 07

Dynamic vs. Static Stretching

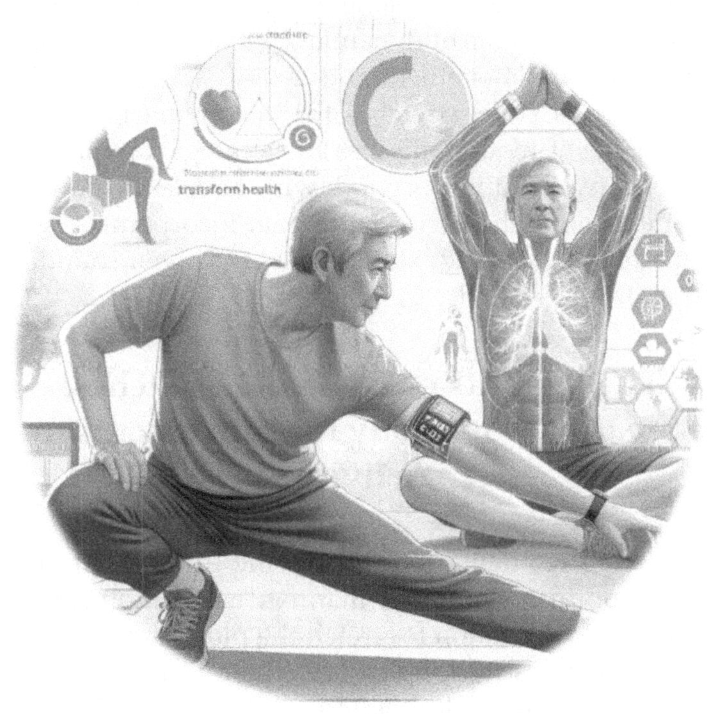

When it comes to flexibility training, there's no shortage of techniques and methods to choose from. However, two of the most common approaches are dynamic and static stretching. In this chapter, we'll explore the benefits of dynamic stretches for preparing your body for movement and activity, delve into the principles of static stretches for improving flexibility and range of motion, discuss the strategic application of each (warm-up vs. cool-down), and learn how to create a comprehensive routine that incorporates both dynamic and static stretches for a well-rounded approach to flexibility training.

The Benefits of Dynamic Stretches: Preparing Your Body for Movement and Activity

Dynamic stretching involves moving through a range of motion in a controlled manner, using momentum and muscle activation to stretch the muscles and joints. Unlike static stretching, which involves holding a stretch for an extended period, dynamic stretches are performed in motion and mimic the movements you'll be doing during your workout or activity.

Dynamic stretches have several benefits, including:

- Increasing blood flow and circulation to the muscles, preparing them for activity.
- Improving flexibility, range of motion, and mobility.
- Enhancing neuromuscular coordination and proprioception.
- Warming up the body and reducing the risk of injury during physical activity.

Incorporating dynamic stretches into your warm-up routine can help prepare your body for movement, improve performance, and reduce the risk of injury during exercise.

Static Stretches Explained: Holding Stretches to Improve Flexibility and Range of Motion

Static stretching involves holding a stretch for a prolonged period (typically 15-60 seconds) without movement. This type of stretching targets specific muscles or muscle groups and aims to improve flexibility, range of motion, and muscle relaxation.

Static stretches have several benefits, including:

- Increasing muscle flexibility and length, allowing for greater range of motion.
- Improving joint mobility and reducing stiffness.
- Promoting relaxation and reducing muscle tension.
- Enhancing overall flexibility and mobility over time.

Static stretches are typically performed after a workout or activity, during the cool-down phase, to help maintain flexibility, prevent muscle soreness, and promote recovery.

Strategic Application: Understanding When to Use Dynamic and Static Stretches (Warm-up vs. Cool-down)

Both dynamic and static stretches have their place in a well-rounded flexibility routine, but understanding when to use each is key to maximizing their effectiveness.

Dynamic stretches are best suited for the warm-up phase of your workout, as they help increase blood flow, activate the muscles, and prepare the body for movement and activity. Performing dynamic stretches before exercise can help improve performance, reduce the risk of injury, and enhance overall readiness for physical activity.

Static stretches, on the other hand, are ideal for the cool-down phase of your workout, as they help relax the muscles, improve flexibility, and promote recovery. Holding static stretches after exercise can help reduce muscle soreness, prevent stiffness, and enhance overall flexibility and mobility over time.

By strategically incorporating both dynamic and static stretches into your flexibility routine, you can optimize your warm-up and cool-down phases, improve performance, reduce the risk of injury, and achieve optimal results from your workouts.

Creating a Comprehensive Routine: Incorporating Both Dynamic and Static Stretches for a Well-Rounded Approach

To create a comprehensive flexibility routine, it's essential to incorporate both dynamic and static stretches into your warm-up and cool-down phases. This ensures that you're adequately preparing your body for movement and activity while also promoting recovery and maintaining flexibility.

Start your routine with 5-10 minutes of dynamic stretches to warm up the muscles, increase blood flow, and prepare the body for exercise. Focus on dynamic movements that target the major muscle groups you'll be using during your workout, such as leg swings, arm circles, and torso twists.

After your workout, spend 10-15 minutes performing static stretches to cool down the muscles, improve flexibility, and promote recovery. Hold each stretch for 15-60 seconds, focusing on major muscle groups such as the hamstrings, quadriceps, calves, chest, shoulders, and back.

By incorporating both dynamic and static stretches into your routine, you can optimize your flexibility training, improve performance, reduce the risk of injury, and achieve optimal results from your workouts.

In summary, dynamic and static stretching each have unique benefits and applications in a flexibility routine. By understanding when to use each type of stretch and strategically incorporating both into your warm-up and cool-down phases, you can optimize your flexibility training and achieve optimal results. With a comprehensive approach to flexibility, you'll enhance performance, reduce the risk of injury, and unlock your body's full potential for movement and activity.

Chapter 08

Upper Body Stretches

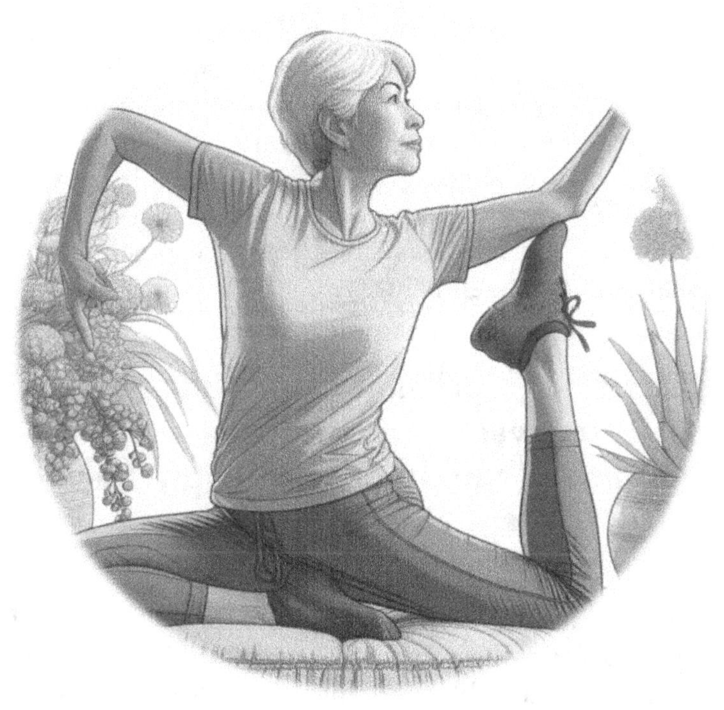

"Tension headaches, rounded shoulders, and tight back muscles — common complaints that plague many of us due to modern lifestyles. But with targeted stretches for the neck, shoulders, and back, you can alleviate discomfort, improve posture, and enhance overall comfort."

In today's sedentary world, many of us spend hours hunched over computers or staring at screens, leading to a host of upper body issues such as neck pain, rounded shoulders, and tight back muscles. In this chapter, we'll address these common complaints head-on, exploring effective stretches to target the neck, shoulders, and back for improved posture and comfort. From gentle stretches for the neck and shoulders to enhancing thoracic spine mobility and promoting a healthy back, you'll discover techniques to alleviate tension headaches, improve posture, and enhance overall well-being.

Addressing Common Upper Body Issues: Effectively Targeting Neck Pain, Rounded Shoulders, and Tight Back Muscles

Modern lifestyles often contribute to a variety of upper body issues, including neck pain, rounded shoulders, and tight back muscles. Addressing these issues requires targeted stretches that release tension, improve flexibility, and promote better alignment.

Neck pain can often be alleviated with gentle stretches that target the neck muscles, such as neck rotations, side bends, and chin tucks. These stretches help release tension, improve range of motion, and reduce stiffness in the neck and upper back.

Rounded shoulders, a common consequence of poor posture and prolonged sitting, can be corrected with stretches that open up the chest and strengthen the muscles of the upper back. Exercises such as doorway stretches, chest openers, and shoulder blade squeezes can help reverse the effects of rounded shoulders and promote better posture.

Tight back muscles, particularly in the thoracic spine, can lead to discomfort and restricted movement. Stretching exercises that target the muscles of the upper back, such as cat-cow stretches, thoracic extensions, and seated twists, can help improve flexibility, mobility, and spinal health.

Gentle Stretches for the Neck and Shoulders: Alleviating Tension Headaches and Improving Posture

Neck and shoulder tension is a common complaint, especially for those who spend long hours sitting at a desk or working on computers. Fortunately, gentle stretches can help alleviate tension headaches, improve posture, and reduce discomfort in the neck and shoulders.

Neck stretches such as the neck side stretch, neck rotation, and neck flexion can help release tension in the neck muscles, improve range of motion, and alleviate headaches caused by muscle tension.

Shoulder stretches such as shoulder rolls, shoulder shrugs, and shoulder blade squeezes can help release tension, improve flexibility, and promote better posture by opening up the chest and strengthening the muscles of the upper back.

Incorporating these gentle stretches into your daily routine can help alleviate neck and shoulder tension, reduce discomfort, and improve overall posture and well-being.

Enhancing Thoracic Spine Mobility: Stretches for Improved Breathing and Spinal Health

The thoracic spine, or upper back, plays a crucial role in posture, breathing, and spinal health. Poor thoracic mobility can lead to stiffness, discomfort, and restricted movement. Fortunately, targeted stretches can help improve thoracic spine mobility and enhance overall well-being.

Thoracic spine stretches such as thoracic extensions, foam roller exercises, and seated twists can help improve flexibility, mobility, and spinal alignment.

These stretches open up the chest, release tension in the upper back muscles, and promote better posture and breathing.

By incorporating thoracic spine stretches into your routine, you can alleviate stiffness, improve mobility, and enhance spinal health for greater comfort and well-being.

Promoting a Healthy Back: Stretches to Prevent and Manage Lower Back Pain

Lower back pain is a common complaint, especially among those who spend long hours sitting or engaging in activities that place stress on the lower back. However, targeted stretches can help prevent and manage lower back pain by improving flexibility, strengthening the core, and promoting better spinal alignment.

Lower back stretches such as the cat-cow stretch, child's pose, and seated spinal twist can help release tension, improve flexibility, and reduce discomfort in the lower back. These stretches lengthen the spine, open up the hips, and promote relaxation in the muscles of the lower back and hips.

Incorporating these stretches into your routine can help prevent lower back pain, alleviate discomfort, and promote a healthy, resilient back for improved comfort and well-being.

In summary, addressing common upper body issues requires targeted stretches that release tension, improve flexibility, and promote better posture and alignment. By incorporating gentle stretches for the neck and shoulders, enhancing thoracic spine mobility, and promoting a healthy back, you can alleviate discomfort, improve posture, and enhance overall well-being for a happier, healthier you.

Chapter 09

Lower Body Stretches

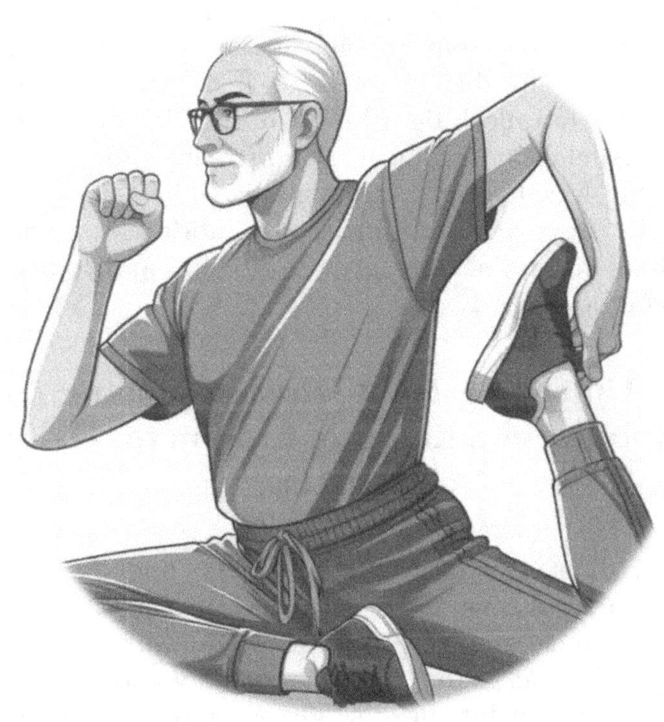

"From tight hips to stiff ankles, our lower body often bears the brunt of daily activities. But with targeted stretches, you can unlock your hips, improve leg flexibility, and maintain healthy feet for better mobility, balance, and overall well-being."

Our lower body is the foundation of movement, yet it's often neglected in our stretching routines. Tight hips, stiff legs, and achy feet are common complaints that can impact our mobility, balance, and overall well-being. In this chapter, we'll explore targeted stretches to unlock tight hips, improve leg flexibility, and maintain healthy feet. From stretches for strong, flexible legs to foot health and flexibility exercises, you'll discover techniques to address specific limitations and achieve greater mobility and comfort in your lower body.

Unlocking Tight Hips: Improving Mobility and Range of Motion for Daily Activities

Tight hips can restrict movement and lead to discomfort during daily activities such as walking, sitting, and bending. Unlocking tight hips requires targeted stretches that improve mobility and range of motion in the hip flexors, glutes, and surrounding muscles.

Hip flexor stretches such as the kneeling hip flexor stretch, pigeon pose, and lunge variations can help release tension and improve flexibility in the front of the hips. These stretches lengthen the hip flexors, open up the hips, and alleviate discomfort associated with tightness.

Glute stretches such as the figure-four stretch, seated piriformis stretch, and supine hip rotation can help release tension and improve flexibility in the glutes and outer hips. These stretches target the muscles of the buttocks and hips, promoting better mobility and comfort.

Incorporating hip stretches into your routine can help improve mobility, reduce discomfort, and enhance overall well-being for greater freedom of movement in daily activities.

Stretches for Strong, Flexible Legs: Maintaining Balance, Coordination, and Agility

Strong, flexible legs are essential for maintaining balance, coordination, and agility in everyday life. Targeted leg stretches can help improve flexibility, range of motion, and strength in the muscles of the legs, thighs, and calves.

Hamstring stretches such as the standing hamstring stretch, seated forward fold, and lying hamstring stretch can help release tension and improve flexibility in the hamstrings. These stretches lengthen the muscles of the back of the thighs, promoting better range of motion and reducing the risk of injury.

Quadriceps stretches such as the standing quad

stretch, kneeling quad stretch, and lying quad stretch can help release tension and improve flexibility in the muscles of the front of the thighs. These stretches target the quadriceps muscles, promoting better mobility and comfort in the legs.

Calf stretches such as the standing calf stretch, wall calf stretch, and seated calf stretch can help release tension and improve flexibility in the calf muscles. These stretches lengthen the muscles of the lower legs, promoting better range of motion and reducing the risk of injury.

Incorporating leg stretches into your routine can help improve flexibility, strength, and mobility in the legs, promoting better balance, coordination, and agility in everyday activities.

Foot Health and Flexibility: Stretches for Plantar Fasciitis Prevention and Improved Balance

Healthy feet are essential for maintaining balance, stability, and overall well-being. Targeted foot stretches can help prevent common foot issues such as plantar fasciitis and improve balance and flexibility in the feet and ankles.

Plantar fascia stretches such as the standing calf stretch with towel, seated foot stretch, and toe stretch can help alleviate tension and improve flexibility in the plantar fascia—the band of tissue that runs along the bottom of the foot. These stretches promote better mobility and reduce the risk of plantar fasciitis and other foot issues.

Ankle stretches such as ankle circles, ankle dorsiflexion stretch, and ankle eversion stretch can help improve flexibility and range of motion in the ankles. These stretches target the muscles and ligaments of the ankles, promoting better balance, stability, and mobility in the feet and ankles.

Incorporating foot stretches into your routine can help prevent foot issues, improve balance, and enhance overall well-being for greater comfort and mobility in daily activities.

Individualized Lower Body Stretching: Tailoring Stretches to Address Specific Limitations

Every body is unique, and individualized stretching routines can help address specific limitations and promote better mobility and comfort in the lower body. Whether you're dealing with tight hips, stiff legs, or achy feet, tailoring stretches to your specific needs can help you achieve greater flexibility and well-being.

Identify areas of tightness or discomfort in your lower body and choose stretches that target those areas. Focus on gentle, controlled movements that gradually lengthen the muscles and promote relaxation and comfort.

Listen to your body's signals and honor its limits, backing off if you feel any sharp or intense pain. With consistency and patience, you can gradually improve flexibility and mobility in your lower body, promoting better balance, comfort, and overall well-being.

In summary, unlocking tight hips, improving leg flexibility, and maintaining healthy feet are essential for greater mobility, balance, and overall well-being. By incorporating targeted stretches into your routine, you can address specific limitations, alleviate discomfort, and achieve greater flexibility and comfort in your lower body for a happier, healthier you.

Chapter 10

Stretching for Specific Needs

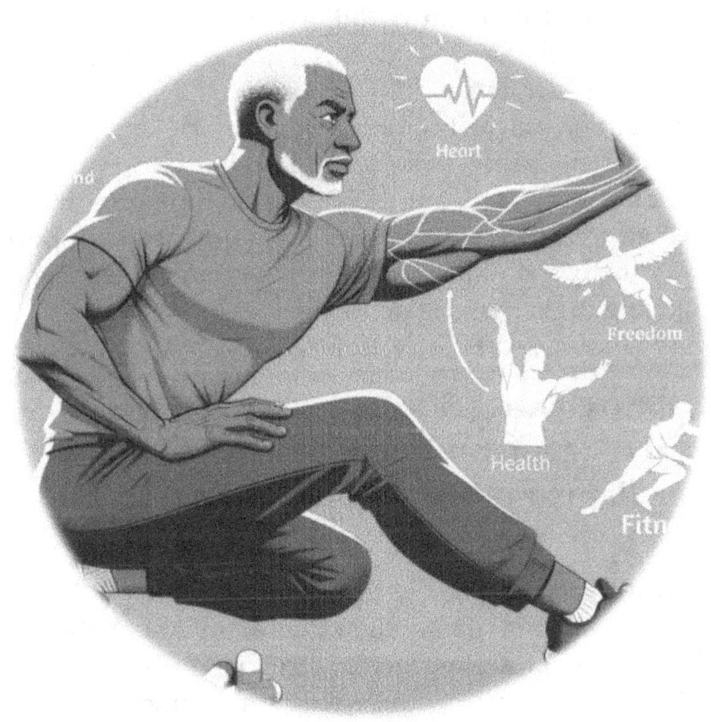

"Stretching isn't just about touching your toes; it's about addressing specific needs and maintaining an active, fulfilling lifestyle. From managing arthritis pain to enhancing balance and stability, optimizing flexibility for sports, and aiding in injury recovery, targeted stretching techniques can support your body's unique requirements and keep you doing what you love."

Stretching isn't a one-size-fits-all solution; it's a versatile tool that can be tailored to address specific needs and challenges. In this chapter, we'll explore stretching strategies for common ailments and maintaining active hobbies. From managing arthritis pain to enhancing balance and stability, optimizing flexibility for sports and hobbies, and aiding in injury recovery, targeted stretching techniques can support your body's unique requirements and keep you enjoying the activities you love.

Stretching Strategies for Arthritis Management: Movement to Alleviate Pain and Improve Joint Function

Arthritis can cause pain, stiffness, and reduced mobility in the joints, making everyday activities challenging. However, gentle stretching exercises can help alleviate pain, improve joint function, and promote better mobility.

Low-impact stretches such as gentle range-of-motion exercises, wrist and hand stretches, and shoulder rolls can help improve flexibility and reduce stiffness in arthritic joints. These stretches should be performed slowly and gently, with a focus on maintaining comfort and avoiding pain.

Incorporating stretching into your daily routine can help manage arthritis symptoms, improve joint function, and enhance overall well-being.

Stretching to Enhance Balance and Stability: Exercises to Improve Fall Prevention and Confidence

Maintaining balance and stability is essential for preventing falls and maintaining independence as we age. Targeted stretching exercises can help improve balance, coordination, and stability, reducing the risk of falls and enhancing confidence in daily activities.

Balance-focused stretches such as tree pose, single-leg stance, and calf raises can help strengthen the muscles of the lower body and improve proprioception—the body's awareness of its position in space. These stretches challenge your balance and stability, promoting better coordination and confidence in your movements.

Incorporating balance-focused stretching exercises into your routine can help improve balance, reduce the risk of falls, and enhance overall confidence and well-being.

Pre- and Post-Activity Stretches: Optimizing Flexibility for Your Favorite Sports and Hobbies

Whether you're an avid runner, cyclist, or golfer, pre- and post-activity stretching can help optimize flexibility, improve performance, and reduce the risk of injury.

Pre-activity stretches such as dynamic warm-up exercises and sport-specific stretches can help prepare your muscles and joints for the demands of your chosen activity. These stretches should be performed before exercise to increase blood flow, improve flexibility, and reduce the risk of injury.

Post-activity stretches such as static stretches and foam rolling can help relax the muscles, reduce soreness, and promote recovery after exercise. These stretches should be performed after exercise to alleviate muscle tension, improve flexibility, and enhance recovery.

Incorporating pre- and post-activity stretching into your routine can help optimize flexibility, improve performance, and reduce the risk of injury during your favorite sports and hobbies.

Stretching for Injury Recovery: Techniques to Promote Healing and a Safe Return to Activity

Injuries are a common occurrence, whether from sports, accidents, or overuse. However, targeted stretching techniques can aid in injury recovery, promote healing, and facilitate a safe return to activity.

Rehabilitation stretches such as gentle range-of-motion exercises, proprioceptive neuromuscular facilitation (PNF) stretches, and mobility exercises can help restore flexibility, strength, and function to injured muscles and joints. These stretches should be performed under the guidance of a healthcare professional and tailored to your specific injury and recovery plan.

Incorporating stretching into your injury recovery program can help promote healing, reduce the risk of re-injury, and facilitate a safe and successful return to activity.

In summary, stretching is a versatile tool that can be tailored to address specific needs and challenges. Whether you're managing arthritis pain, improving balance and stability, optimizing flexibility for sports and hobbies, or recovering from injury, targeted stretching techniques can support your body's unique requirements and keep you doing what you love. By incorporating stretching into your routine, you can enhance mobility, reduce pain, and maintain an active, fulfilling lifestyle for years to come.

Part 4:
Living a Life Filled with Movement

Chapter 11

Movement Beyond the Mat

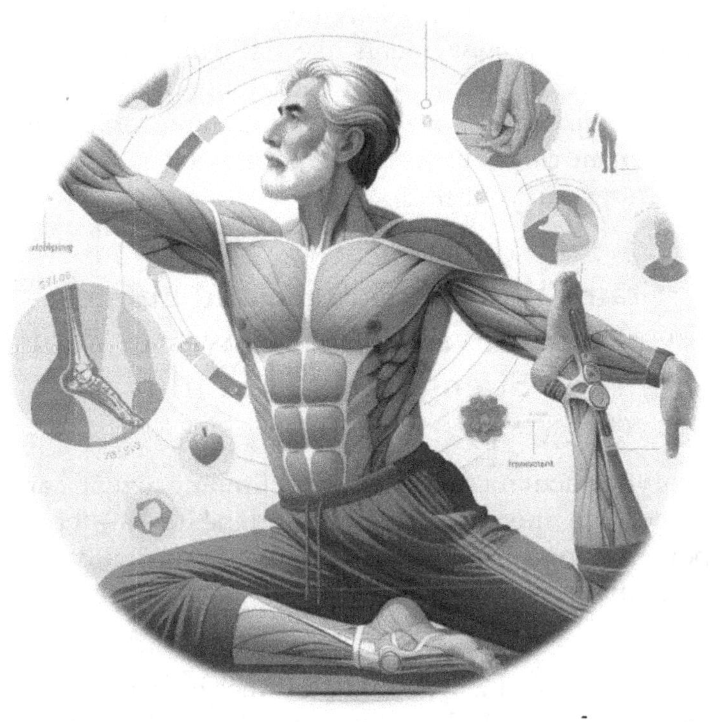

"Movement isn't just confined to the gym—it's woven into the fabric of our daily lives. From stair climbing to gardening, dance classes to group fitness, embracing functional activities can transform mundane tasks into opportunities for strength, flexibility, joy, and community."

Movement is not just a structured activity confined to the walls of a gym; it's an integral part of our daily lives. In this chapter, we'll explore the power of integrating functional activities into your routine. From everyday movements like stair climbing, squats, and lunges to finding joy in gardening, dance classes, and group fitness, we'll delve into how embracing movement can enhance strength, flexibility, joy, and community in your life.

Stair Climbing, Squats, and Lunges: Everyday Movements as Powerful Tools for Strength and Flexibility

Everyday activities such as stair climbing, squats, and lunges are more than just mundane tasks—they're powerful tools for improving strength, flexibility, and mobility.

Stair climbing engages multiple muscle groups in the lower body, including the quadriceps, hamstrings, glutes, and calves, while also providing a cardiovascular workout. Incorporating stair climbing into your daily routine can help improve lower body strength, endurance, and flexibility.

Squats and lunges are functional movements that mimic everyday activities like sitting down and standing up. These exercises target the muscles of the legs, hips, and core, promoting better balance, stability, and mobility. By incorporating squats and lunges into your routine, you can improve lower body strength, flexibility, and overall functional fitness.

Gardening with Intention: Turning Yard Work into a Functional Mobility Workout

Gardening isn't just a hobby—it's also a fantastic way to incorporate movement into your daily routine and improve functional mobility.

Activities like digging, planting, and weeding engage muscles throughout the body, promoting strength, flexibility, and endurance. By approaching gardening with intention and mindfulness, you can turn yard work into a functional mobility workout that improves overall fitness and well-being.

Incorporate dynamic movements like squatting, bending, reaching, and lifting to engage different muscle groups and promote better mobility and flexibility. Take breaks to stretch and hydrate, and listen to your body's signals to avoid overexertion and injury.

Dance Classes and Group Fitness: The Joy of Movement and the Power of Community

Dance classes and group fitness offer more than just physical benefits—they also provide opportunities for joy, expression, and community.

Dancing engages the body and mind in a dynamic and expressive way, promoting cardiovascular health, coordination, flexibility, and emotional well-being. Whether you prefer salsa, hip-hop, or ballroom dancing, there's a dance style for everyone to enjoy.

Group fitness classes such as yoga, Pilates, and Zumba offer a supportive and motivating environment to exercise and connect with others. These classes provide a variety of movements and intensity levels to accommodate different fitness levels and preferences.

Finding Activities You Love: Making Movement a Source of Enjoyment and Motivation

The key to sustaining a regular movement practice is finding activities that you enjoy and that align with your interests and goals.

Experiment with different forms of movement—

whether it's hiking, cycling, swimming, or rock climbing—to discover what brings you joy and fulfillment. Consider joining clubs, teams, or classes to connect with like-minded individuals and find motivation and support.

Remember that movement is not just about achieving a specific fitness goal; it's about enjoying the journey and embracing the process. By finding activities you love, you can make movement a sustainable and rewarding part of your daily life.

In summary, movement is not confined to the gym—it's woven into the fabric of our daily lives. By embracing functional activities like stair climbing, gardening, dance classes, and group fitness, you can improve strength, flexibility, joy, and community in your life. Find activities you love, make movement a source of enjoyment and motivation, and discover the transformative power of integrating movement into your daily routine.

Chapter 12

Building Strength & Balance

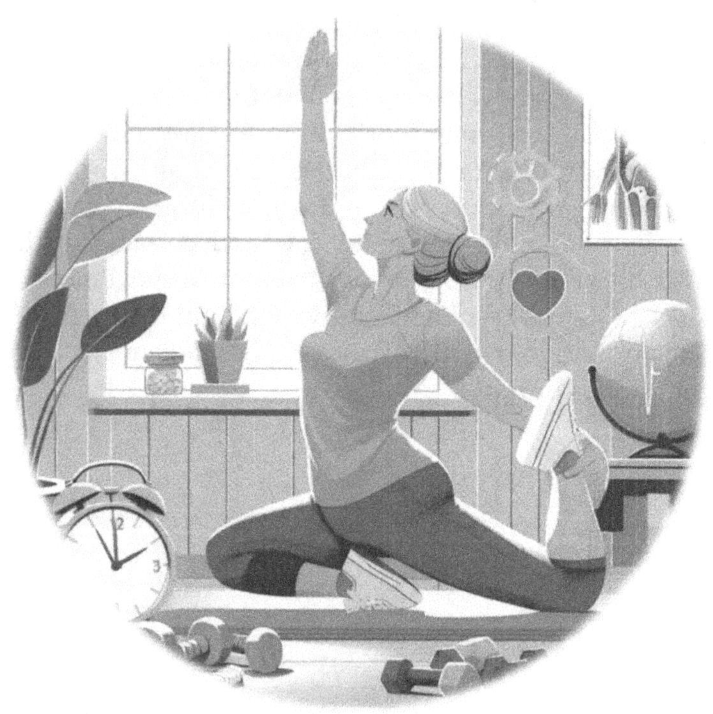

"Strength and balance are the pillars of independence as we age. By incorporating simple balance training techniques and effective strength-building exercises into your routine, you can enhance stability, prevent falls, and build the strength needed for a strong and independent future."

As we age, maintaining strength and balance becomes increasingly important for preserving independence and quality of life. In this chapter, we'll explore a variety of exercises designed to improve strength and balance, including simple balance training techniques, bodyweight exercises, strength training tools for home, and strategies for progression and modification. By incorporating these exercises into your routine, you can enhance stability, prevent falls, and build the strength needed for a strong and independent future.

Balance Training Techniques: Simple Exercises to Improve Stability and Prevent Falls

Balance is a key component of functional fitness and plays a crucial role in preventing falls and maintaining independence. Incorporating simple balance training techniques into your routine can improve stability and reduce the risk of falls.

Balance exercises such as single-leg stands, heel-to-toe walks, and balance board exercises challenge your stability and proprioception—the body's sense of its position in space. These exercises strengthen the muscles of the lower body and core, improve balance, and enhance coordination and confidence in movement.

Incorporate balance exercises into your routine several times a week to improve stability, prevent falls, and maintain independence as you age.

Building Strength with Bodyweight Exercises: Effective Exercises that Require No Equipment

Strength training is essential for maintaining muscle mass, bone density, and overall functional fitness as we age. Bodyweight exercises are a convenient and effective way to build strength without the need for equipment.

Exercises such as squats, lunges, push-ups, and planks target multiple muscle groups simultaneously, promoting strength, stability, and endurance. These exercises can be modified to suit your fitness level and performed anywhere, making them ideal for home workouts or when traveling.

Incorporate bodyweight exercises into your routine two to three times a week to build strength, improve mobility, and enhance overall functional fitness.

Strength Training Tools for Home: Utilizing Resistance Bands, Free Weights, or Household Items to Build Strength

While bodyweight exercises are effective for building strength, incorporating additional resistance can further challenge your muscles and promote greater gains. Resistance bands, free weights, or household items can be used to add resistance to your strength training routine.

Resistance bands are versatile and portable, making them ideal for home workouts. They can be used to perform a variety of exercises targeting the upper and lower body, such as bicep curls, rows, and leg lifts.

Free weights, such as dumbbells or kettlebells, provide added resistance and can be used to perform a wide range of strength training exercises, including squats, lunges, chest presses, and shoulder raises.

Household items such as water bottles, canned goods, or bags of rice can also be used as improvised weights for strength training exercises.

Incorporate resistance training into your routine two to three times a week to build strength, improve muscle tone, and enhance overall functional fitness.

Progression and Modification: Adapting Exercises to Your Fitness Level and Ensuring Safe Progress

Progression and modification are key principles of effective strength training. By gradually increasing the intensity of your workouts and adapting exercises to your fitness level, you can ensure safe progress and avoid plateaus.

Start with exercises that challenge your current fitness level, focusing on proper form and technique. As you become stronger, gradually increase the intensity of your workouts by adding more resistance, increasing repetitions, or performing advanced variations of exercises.

Listen to your body's signals and avoid pushing yourself too hard or too fast. If an exercise causes pain or discomfort, modify it or seek guidance from a qualified fitness professional.

By incorporating progression and modification into your strength training routine, you can safely build strength, improve muscle tone, and enhance overall functional fitness for a strong and independent future.

In summary, building strength and balance are essential components of maintaining independence and quality of life as we age. By incorporating simple balance training techniques, bodyweight exercises, strength training tools for home, and strategies for progression and modification into your routine, you can enhance stability, prevent falls, and build the strength needed for a strong and independent future. Start slowly, listen to your body, and enjoy the benefits of a stronger, more resilient body for years to come.

Chapter 13

Mindfulness & Movement

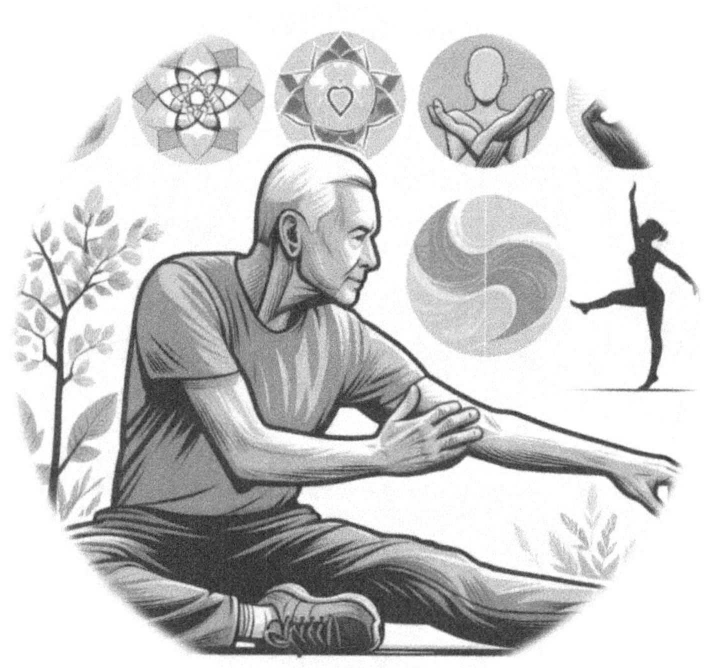

In this final chapter, we embark on a profound exploration of the intersection between mindfulness and movement. We'll delve deeper into the techniques that not only foster flexibility and strength but also cultivate a resilient mindset and inner peace. By intertwining mindfulness with our physical practice, we unlock the potential for holistic wellness and a richer, more fulfilling life.

The Power of Breathwork: Utilizing Mindful Breathing Techniques to Enhance Stretching and Manage Stress

Breath is the bridge between mind and body, and harnessing its power can profoundly enhance our physical and mental well-being. Mindful breathing techniques provide a pathway to relaxation, stress reduction, and deeper stretching.

Begin by finding a comfortable seated or lying position, allowing your body to relax and your breath to become natural. Bring your awareness to the sensation of your breath entering and leaving your body, noticing the rise and fall of your chest and belly.

As you begin to stretch, synchronize your breath with your movements, inhaling deeply as you lengthen and exhaling fully as you release tension. Use your breath as a guide, allowing it to lead you deeper into each stretch and promote a sense of ease and openness.

Practice deep diaphragmatic breathing, focusing on slow, rhythmic inhales and exhales that fill your belly with air. This type of breathing activates the body's relaxation response, reducing stress hormones and promoting a sense of calm and well-being.

Incorporate breathwork into your stretching routine to enhance flexibility, release tension, and cultivate a deeper connection between mind and body. By harnessing the power of breath, you can optimize your stretching practice and unlock greater levels of relaxation and ease.

The Connection Between Body and Mind: Cultivating Body Awareness and a Positive Self-Image

In a world that often emphasizes external appearance over internal strength, cultivating body awareness is a radical act of self-love and acceptance. By tuning into the sensations of our body during movement, we deepen our connection with ourselves and foster a positive self-image.

Practice mindful movement by bringing your attention to the present moment, noticing the sensations of stretching, contracting, and releasing muscles. Allow yourself to become fully immersed in the experience of movement, letting go of judgment and expectations.

As you stretch, pay attention to the messages your body is sending you. Notice areas of tension or discomfort and adjust your movements accordingly, honoring your body's needs and boundaries.

Cultivate a positive self-image by focusing on what your body can do rather than its appearance. Celebrate its strength, resilience, and capacity for growth, recognizing that true beauty comes from within.

Visualizations for Enhanced Results: Using Mental Imagery to Optimize Your Stretching Practice

The mind is a powerful tool that can be harnessed to enhance the effectiveness of our stretching practice. By engaging in mental imagery and visualization techniques, we can optimize our body's response to stretching and achieve greater levels of flexibility and relaxation.

Begin by setting an intention for your stretching practice, visualizing the outcomes you wish to achieve and the sensations you hope to experience. Imagine yourself performing each stretch with ease and grace, envisioning your muscles lengthening and releasing tension with each breath.

Use imagery to create a mental blueprint for your practice, focusing on positive affirmations that reinforce your ability to stretch and grow. Visualize yourself overcoming challenges and achieving your goals, cultivating a mindset of confidence and possibility.

As you stretch, use mental imagery to deepen your connection with your body and enhance the effectiveness of each movement. Imagine the sensation of warmth and openness spreading throughout your body as you deepen into each stretch, allowing yourself to relax and let go.

By incorporating visualizations into your stretching practice, you can optimize your body's response to stretching, deepen your connection with yourself, and achieve greater levels of flexibility and relaxation.

Building Resilience Through Movement: Developing a Growth Mindset and Celebrating Small Victories

Movement is not just about physical fitness—it's also a powerful tool for building resilience and developing a growth mindset. By embracing the journey of movement, celebrating small victories, and learning from setbacks, we cultivate inner strength and resilience that extends far beyond the mat.

Approach your movement practice with a sense of curiosity and openness, viewing challenges as opportunities for growth and learning. Embrace the process of stretching and strengthening your body, knowing that each step forward brings you closer to your goals.

Celebrate small victories along the way, whether it's

touching your toes for the first time or holding a challenging stretch for an extra few seconds. Acknowledge your progress and give yourself credit for the effort you've put in, recognizing that every step forward is a testament to your resilience and determination.

Use setbacks as opportunities for reflection and growth, learning from your experiences and adjusting your approach as needed. Cultivate a growth mindset that embraces challenges and sees failure as a stepping stone to success.

By embracing the journey of movement, developing a growth mindset, and celebrating small victories, we build resilience and inner strength that empower us to face life's challenges with confidence and grace.

Conclusion: Embracing Mindfulness and Movement for a Fulfilling Life

In the fast-paced world we live in, it's easy to lose sight of the connection between mind and body. Yet, by embracing mindfulness and movement, we unlock the potential for holistic wellness and a richer, more fulfilling life.

Through mindful breathing techniques, we enhance our ability to relax, reduce stress, and deepen our stretching practice. By cultivating body awareness and a positive self-image, we foster a deeper connection with ourselves and promote self-love and acceptance. Through visualizations and mental imagery, we optimize our body's response to stretching and achieve greater levels of flexibility and relaxation. And by embracing a growth mindset and celebrating small victories, we build resilience and inner strength that empower us to face life's challenges with confidence and grace.

As we embark on this journey of mindfulness and movement, may we find joy in the present moment, strength in our bodies, and peace in our hearts. May we honor the sacred connection between mind and body and embrace the transformative power of movement to lead lives filled with vitality, purpose, and fulfillment.

Part 5:
Maintaining Motivation & Living Your Best Life

Chapter 14

Sustainable
Stretching Habits

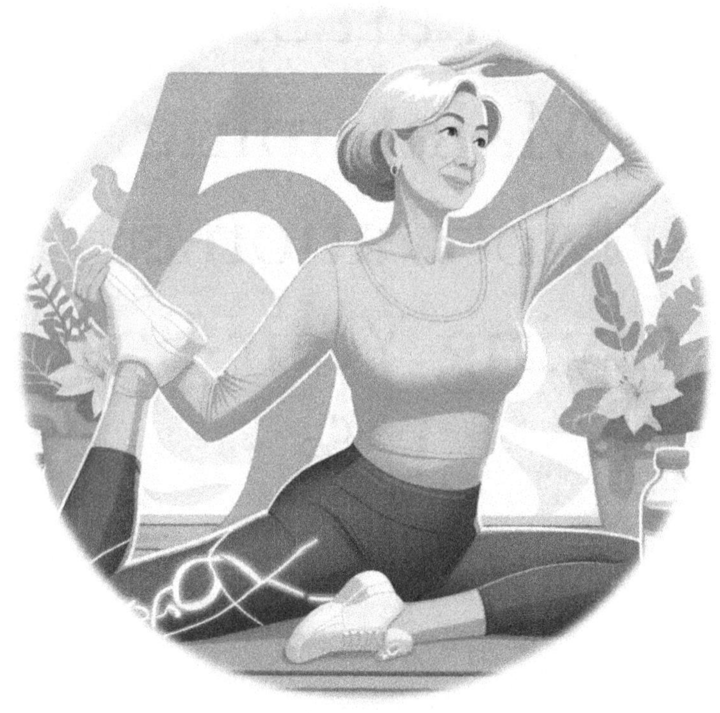

"Building a sustainable stretching habit isn't just about occasional bursts of effort—it's about consistent, long-term commitment. In this chapter, we'll explore effective strategies and practical tips to help you establish a lasting stretching routine that supports your health and well-being well into the future."

Establishing a sustainable stretching habit requires more than just sporadic efforts; it demands consistent commitment and dedication. In this chapter, we'll delve into effective strategies and practical tips to help you cultivate a lasting stretching routine that nurtures your health and well-being for years to come.

Setting SMART Stretching Goals: Creating Clear, Achievable Goals to Stay Motivated

Setting clear and achievable goals is the first step towards building a sustainable stretching habit. By using the SMART criteria—specific, measurable, achievable, relevant, and time-bound—you can create goals that are meaningful and motivating.

Define specific stretching goals that align with your overall health and wellness objectives. Whether it's improving flexibility, reducing pain, or enhancing mobility, clarity is key to staying focused and motivated.

Ensure your goals are measurable, allowing you to

track your progress and celebrate small victories along the way. This could involve measuring your range of motion, tracking the duration of your stretches, or noting improvements in how you feel.

Make sure your goals are achievable, considering your current level of flexibility, time constraints, and other commitments. Setting unrealistic goals can lead to frustration and demotivation, so be realistic about what you can accomplish.

Ensure your goals are relevant to your overall health and well-being, aligning with your values and priorities. When your goals are personally meaningful, you're more likely to stay committed and motivated over the long term.

Finally, set time-bound goals with specific deadlines or milestones to keep you accountable and focused. Breaking your goals down into smaller, manageable tasks can help prevent overwhelm and maintain momentum.

By setting SMART stretching goals, you can create a roadmap for success and stay motivated on your journey to improved flexibility and mobility.

Tracking Your Progress: Monitoring Improvement and Celebrating Milestones to Stay Engaged

Monitoring your progress is essential for staying

motivated and maintaining momentum in your stretching routine. By tracking your improvement and celebrating milestones, you can stay engaged and inspired to continue making progress.

Keep a stretching journal or use a tracking app to record your stretching sessions, noting the duration, intensity, and any changes in flexibility or mobility. This allows you to see how far you've come and identify areas for improvement.

Take regular measurements of your range of motion or flexibility using simple tests or assessments. Tracking your progress over time provides tangible evidence of your improvement and reinforces your commitment to your stretching routine.

Celebrate milestones along the way, whether it's touching your toes for the first time, increasing your range of motion, or reducing pain and discomfort. Acknowledge your achievements and give yourself credit for the effort you've put in.

Share your progress with friends, family, or your stretching community for added accountability and support. Celebrating your successes with others can boost your motivation and inspire others to join you on your journey.

By tracking your progress and celebrating milestones, you can stay engaged and motivated in your stretching routine, fueling your progress and momentum over the long term.

Overcoming Plateaus: Identifying and Addressing Challenges to Maintain Progress

Plateaus are a natural part of any fitness journey, but they can be frustrating and demotivating if not addressed effectively. By identifying and addressing the challenges that contribute to plateaus, you can maintain progress and keep moving forward in your stretching routine.

Evaluate your stretching routine and look for areas where you may have become stagnant or complacent. Are you consistently challenging yourself and varying your stretches, or have you fallen into a rut? Identifying areas for improvement is the first step towards overcoming plateaus.

Experiment with new stretching techniques, exercises, or routines to keep your body guessing and prevent adaptation. Introduce variety into your stretching routine by incorporating different stretches, props, or modalities to target different muscle groups and movement patterns.

Focus on quality over quantity in your stretching sessions, ensuring proper form and technique to maximize effectiveness and prevent injury. Slow down and pay attention to your body's signals, avoiding the temptation to rush through your stretches or push past your limits.

Consider incorporating cross-training or complementary activities into your routine to address imbalances and enhance overall flexibility and mobility. Activities like yoga, Pilates, or tai chi can complement your stretching routine and provide additional benefits for physical and mental well-being.

By addressing plateaus head-on and implementing strategies to overcome challenges, you can maintain progress and momentum in your stretching routine, ensuring continued growth and improvement over time.

Building a Support System: Finding a Community or Accountability Partner for Encouragement

Building a support system is essential for staying motivated and accountable in your stretching routine. Whether it's joining a stretching class, finding a workout buddy, or connecting with an online community, having support and encouragement can make all the difference in staying committed to your goals.

Join a stretching class or group in your community to connect with like-minded individuals and find motivation and support. Participating in group sessions provides accountability and camaraderie, making your stretching routine more enjoyable and sustainable.

Find a workout buddy or accountability partner to share your stretching journey with and keep each other motivated and on track. Whether it's a friend, family member, or colleague, having someone to share your progress with can boost your motivation and commitment.

Connect with an online stretching community or forum to find support and inspiration from people around the world who share your goals and challenges. Engaging with others who are on a similar journey can provide encouragement, advice, and motivation to keep pushing forward.

By building a support system of friends, family, or fellow stretching enthusiasts, you can stay motivated and accountable in your stretching routine, ensuring consistency and long-term success.

Conclusion: Embracing a Lifetime of Health and Wellness

In the journey towards health and wellness, consistency is key. By creating a sustainable stretching habit and incorporating effective strategies for long-term success, you can cultivate a lifetime of flexibility, mobility, and vitality.

Set SMART stretching goals that are specific, measurable, achievable, relevant, and time-bound to stay focused and motivated on your journey. Track your progress, celebrate milestones, and share your successes with others to stay engaged and inspired.

Overcome plateaus by identifying and addressing challenges, experimenting with new techniques, and incorporating variety into your routine. And build a support system of friends, family, or fellow stretching enthusiasts to stay motivated and accountable on your path to health and wellness.

By embracing these tips and strategies for creating a sustainable stretching habit, you can maintain flexibility, mobility, and well-being well into the future, ensuring a lifetime of health and vitality. Here's to living your best life after 50 and beyond!

Chapter 15

Embrace Your Active Life

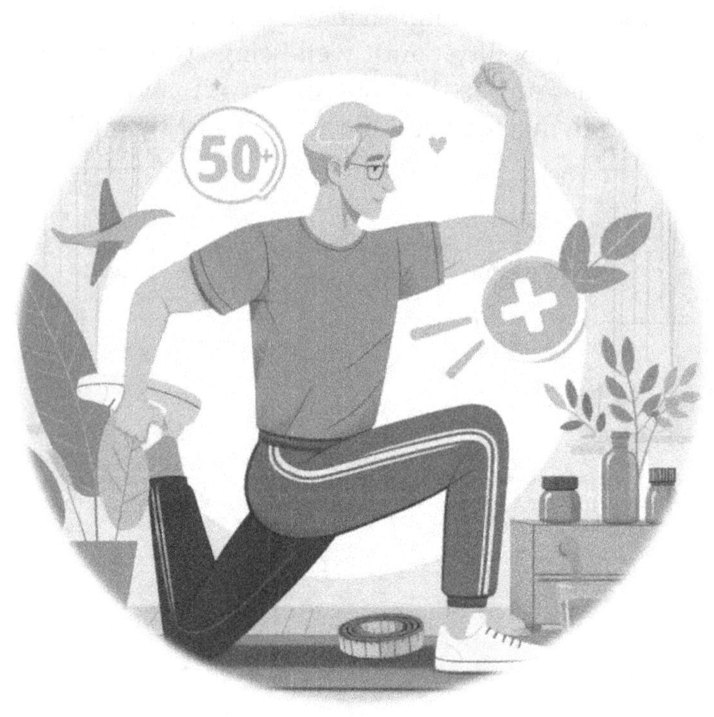

Life after 50 is a journey filled with boundless opportunities for growth, exploration, and fulfillment. In this final chapter, we embark on a journey of self-discovery and empowerment, exploring how to embrace an active life with confidence and flexibility, celebrating the resilience of your body and the vitality of your spirit.

Living a Life Without Limits: Exploring New Activities and Adventures with a Flexible Body and a Strong Spirit

As we age, it's easy to fall into the trap of self-imposed limitations, believing that our bodies are no longer capable of the activities and adventures we once enjoyed. However, with a flexible body and a strong spirit, the possibilities for exploration and adventure are endless.

Challenge yourself to step outside your comfort zone and try new activities and adventures that ignite your passion and curiosity. Whether it's hiking, dancing, kayaking, or learning a new sport, embrace the opportunity to explore and discover new experiences.

Approach each new adventure with a sense of

openness and enthusiasm, knowing that your flexible body and strong spirit are more than capable of rising to the challenge. Trust in your abilities and believe in your potential to thrive in every aspect of life, regardless of age.

By living a life without limits and embracing new activities and adventures with a flexible body and a strong spirit, you can unlock a world of possibilities and experience a newfound sense of vitality and joy.

Prioritizing Rest and Recovery: Listening to Your Body to Prevent Burnout and Optimize Results

While staying active and engaged is important for overall health and well-being, it's equally essential to prioritize rest and recovery to prevent burnout and optimize results. Listening to your body and honoring its need for rest is key to maintaining balance and longevity in your active lifestyle.

Recognize the signs of overexertion and fatigue, such as persistent soreness, decreased performance, and difficulty sleeping. When you notice these signs, take a step back and give your body the rest and recovery it needs to rejuvenate and repair.

Incorporate restorative activities such as gentle stretching, meditation, or leisurely walks into your routine to promote relaxation and recovery. These activities not only help to alleviate physical tension but also calm the mind and reduce stress, enhancing overall well-being.

Remember that rest and recovery are essential components of any successful fitness regimen. By prioritizing rest and listening to your body's cues, you can prevent burnout, optimize results, and sustain your active lifestyle for the long term.

The Ageless Mindset: Embracing Your Age and Celebrating the Power of Your Body

Age is just a number, and the key to living with confidence and flexibility over 50 lies in embracing an ageless mindset. Rather than viewing age as a limitation, see it as a badge of honor—a testament to the wisdom, resilience, and strength you've gained over the years.

Celebrate your age and the unique journey that has brought you to this moment. Embrace the wrinkles, scars, and imperfections as symbols of a life well-lived and experiences cherished. Recognize that true beauty comes from within and radiates from a spirit that is alive with vitality and joy.

Focus on what your body can do rather than its limitations, celebrating its strength, resilience, and capacity for growth. Approach each day with gratitude and appreciation for the gift of movement and the opportunity to live life to the fullest.

By embracing an ageless mindset and celebrating the power of your body, you can cultivate a sense of confidence and vitality that transcends age. Embrace the journey of aging with grace and resilience, knowing that the best is yet to come.

Stretching Strong: A Legacy for a Vibrant and Fulfilling Life After 50

As we conclude our journey of embracing an active life with confidence and flexibility over 50, remember that the legacy you leave is not measured by the years you've lived but by the lives you've touched and the memories you've created. By stretching strong and living with intention, you can inspire others to embrace their own journey of health and vitality.

Share your passion for movement and wellness with those around you, encouraging them to prioritize their health and well-being at every age. Lead by example, embodying the principles of flexibility, resilience, and joy in everything you do.

As you continue on your path, remember that the journey of life is not a sprint but a marathon—a journey of growth, exploration, and self-discovery. Embrace each day with enthusiasm and curiosity, knowing that your flexible body and strong spirit are capable of achieving anything you set your mind to.

In closing, may you continue to embrace your active life with confidence and flexibility, celebrating the strength of your body and the power of your spirit. Here's to living life to the fullest, embracing every opportunity with open arms, and stretching strong for a vibrant and fulfilling life after 50.

CONCLUSION

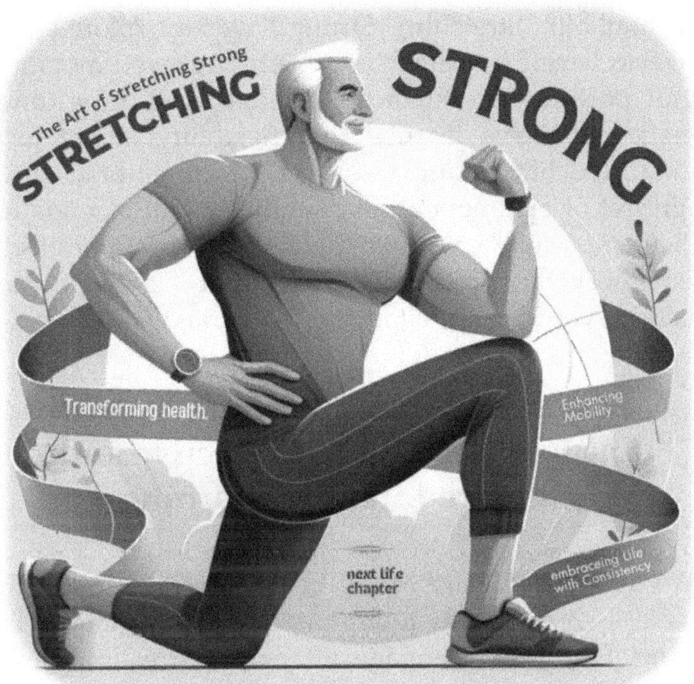

As we reach the conclusion of our journey together, it's time to reflect on the transformative power of flexibility in your life and reaffirm your commitment to continued growth and well-being. In this final stretch, let's recap key takeaways, renew our commitment to growth, inspire others to join the journey, and celebrate the incredible potential that lies within each of us.

Recap of Key Takeaways: A Final Look at the Transformative Power of Flexibility in Your Life

Throughout "Stretching Strong," we've explored the myriad benefits of flexibility, from improved mobility and posture to enhanced mental well-being and resilience. We've learned that flexibility is not just about touching your toes—it's about embracing a mindset of openness and adaptability that extends to all areas of life. As we take this final moment to reflect, remember the profound impact that flexibility can have on your health, vitality, and overall well-being.

A Commitment to Continued Growth: Encouragement to Stay Active and Embrace Lifelong Learning

As you reach the end of this book, I encourage you to make a commitment to continued growth and well-being. Stay active, engage in regular stretching and exercise, and embrace opportunities for lifelong learning and personal development. Whether it's trying a new activity, exploring a new hobby, or deepening your understanding of health and wellness, never stop seeking out new experiences and challenges that enrich your life and expand your horizons.

Sharing Your Journey: Inspiring Others to Take Charge of Their Well-being Through Stretching

As you continue on your journey of health and vitality, remember that you have the power to inspire and empower others to take charge of their own well-being. Share your experiences, insights, and successes with friends, family, and your community, and encourage them to join you in embracing the transformative power of stretching. By leading by example and sharing your journey, you can create a ripple effect of positive change that extends far beyond yourself.

The Final Stretch: A Concluding Message of Empowerment and a Celebration of Your Potential

In this final stretch, I want to leave you with a message of empowerment and celebration. You have embarked on a journey of self-discovery and transformation, and you have the power to shape your own destiny and create the vibrant, fulfilling life you deserve. Believe in yourself, trust in your abilities, and never underestimate the incredible potential that lies within you. As you continue on your journey, know that you are capable of achieving anything you set your mind to, and that the best is yet to come.

Conclusion: Embrace the Last Stretch and Step Into Your Bright Future

In closing, I want to thank you for joining me on this journey of exploration and growth. As you embrace the last stretch and step into your bright future, remember that the power to create the life you desire lies within you. With flexibility as your guide and empowerment as your fuel, there's no limit to what you can achieve. So, take a deep breath, stretch strong, and step boldly into the next chapter of your journey. Your future is waiting—and it's filled with endless possibilities.

www.ingramcontent.com/pod-product-compliance
Lightning Source LLC
Chambersburg PA
CBHW081522250726
48659CB00009B/2905